THE NATURE CURE TREATMENT FOR VARICOSE VEINS AND ULCERS

Varicose veins, varicose ulcers, haemorrhoids and phlebitis are all complaints directly arising from breakdown of the circulatory tissues. Injections and surgical removal can offer nothing more than temporary alleviation. In this book an experienced Nature Cure practitioner explains the causes of breakdown and provides self-treatment methods by which the resultant disorders may be permanently overcome.

The Nature Cure Treatment for Varicose Veins and Ulcers

J. Russell Sneddon N.D., M.B.N.O.A.

THORSONS PUBLISHERS LIMITED
Wellingborough, Northamptonshire

First published 1950
Tenth Impression 1971
Second Edition, revised and reset, 1974
Second Impression 1977
Third Impression 1979
Fourth Impression 1980
Fifth Impression 1982

ISBN 0 7225 0269 9 (paperback)
ISBN 0 7225 0357 1 (hardback)

Printed in Great Britain by
Richard Clay (The Chaucer Press) Ltd,
Bungay, Suffolk

Contents

Introduction

Viewed from many angles it would appear that modern man has made a sorry mess of his world. On every hand it becomes apparent that, although the struggle to penetrate the secrets of the universe has been frequently successful, most of the knowledge gained has been utilized to satisfy the demand for power and greed, envy and jealousy, of men and nations.

It is clear to thinking men and women that it does not pay to antagonize nature by robbing her and then using the gained information against her. We have the intelligence to gain power but seemingly cannot use it in harmony with nature. Yet it is only by working with, and not against, nature that we gain health of mind and body and fulfil our proper function in this life.

This book has been written from the viewpoint of a Nature Cure practitioner, and we believe that by obeying nature's laws in so far as is possible in a modern world we can avoid many of the common physical ailments. We also believe that immediately a person suffering from any complaint stops breaking natural law he starts to get well, the amount of recovery being limited only by the strength of his will and the power in his cells.

It is from this angle, that of working in accordance with the dictates of nature, that I wish to explain the sensible methods of treating all kinds of vein weakness.

Varicosity of the veins means that these blood vessels, which are used to return unclean blood to the heart and are, in normal health, unseen, dilate and appear on the surface of the skin as soft bluish dwellings. The swellings disappear on light pressure and when the sufferer is lying down, but even then it is possible to feel hardish lumps and knots along the course of seriously damaged vessels.

This trouble affects the veins rather than the arteries because the former, although similar in construction, are lacking in an elastic coat and are therefore more liable to injury. Again, the veins carry dirty blood, and if this blood contains some undesirable impurity it is likely to get lodged in one of the valves and cause inflammation. The arteries, on the other hand, deal with cleansed blood, and if this is in a normal condition there is not the same tendency for inflammation to arise.

Generally the veins of the lower trunk and limbs are chiefly affected, but the trouble can be found in any part of the body supplied with these vessels, and there can be internal varicosity in certain parts. The reason for the prevalence of varicosity in the lower limbs lies in the mechanics of the body's circulation, which are roughly as follows.

Venous blood from the feet is not pumped back to the heart but is forced upwards by the relaxation and contraction of the muscles surrounding the veins. As the blood flows towards the heart it is prevented from obeying the law of gravity and falling downwards again by small non-return valves placed every inch or so along the course of the veins. These valves, not needed in the more elastic arteries, provide weak spots in vein construction, because it is here that inflammation always arises. This inflammation, in serious conditions, is called phlebitis, but in the beginning of varicosity it is slight enough to pass unnoticed and must not be confused with an actual severe attack of this trouble. The usual result of these minor inflammations is that one or more valves are completely destroyed and a certain length of the vein is subjected to increased venous pressure.

Because the vein is normally lacking in elastic tissue it weakens under this extra strain and swells and dilates until it assumes the well-known appearance of varicosity.

Swelling and knotting of the superficial veins of the abdomen and lower extremities quickly lead to unsightliness, and it is often this factor alone that causes the sufferer to seek advice. In many cases this is a decided advantage, because it results in early treatment and the trouble is checked before it reaches serious proportions.

GNAWING TIREDNESS

Most sufferers, however, appreciate the change in the condition of their veins but are content to carry on without treatment because they do not feel any great discomfort. Discomfort does come eventually, and usually it takes the form of a gnawing tiredness, which makes the working hours of the sufferer a misery and which may be only slightly relieved during rest. Such an intense tiredness affects all the patient's life, because it cannot be alleviated to any great extent, and naturally the general health suffers and a great deal of the attractiveness of life is lost.

Breakage in the venous system is always serious because it is progressive and can lead to a lifetime of misery. Early treatment can be most effective, and the system outlined in this book will aid every case of varicosity and will provide a complete cure in many cases.

The untreated condition is always getting worse because of the mechanics of the disability. When one part of the vein wall collapses more strain is placed on the adjacent parts and they in turn become quickly affected. Each month that is allowed to elapse without treatment means that so many more inches of the vein become weakened, and it must be stressed that once the vein wall becomes seriously affected no regeneration of the part is possible, although the pain and tiredness may be removed.

Varicosity of the veins is always potentially danger-ous because a small piece of a broken valve inside the vein wall may become detached and carried through the circulation to a vital part of the body. Here it may choke one of the more important arteries or else cause heart block. Irreparable damage can follow this temporary or permanent blockage of an artery.

Phlebitis, a serious inflammation of the veins, usually the leg, is a condition that arises readily in a part already affected by varicosity. Injection treat-ment for varicosity often results in phlebitis, and this is one of the reasons why this practice is not advised in every case, although this treatment may be of benefit after a course of Nature Cure.

CAUSE OF VARICOSE ULCER

Again, varicosity is always dangerous because, if allowed to continue for an indefinite period, it results in poor circulation of the skin around the part affected. This usually occurs in the lower extremities. In time the skin of this part weakens and, if the blood becomes dirty, the usual result is breakage of the skin surface, forming a varicose ulcer.

These ulcers, because they act as artificial drains for the impure blood stream, are difficult to heal, and many people have spent much time and money trying to get a cure for such conditions. In passing it may be stated that nearly all the treatment advised for varicose ulcers is of a suppressive nature, and this fact accounts for the poor results in such treatment. In this book the modern eliminative method of treating varicose ulcers is carefully outlined, and it will be found that it is most successful.

In varicosity there is a very real danger of thinning of the vein wall with the result that even a light abrasion may result in excessive bleeding in a pin-point wound. The blood in such cases comes away in a very fine spray, and a great deal can be lost before the patient becomes aware of the wound, especially if he or she is sleeping at the time.

It follows that every sufferer from varicose veins must be most careful to avoid injury to these parts. Even a brisk rubbing with a rough towel has been known to break the outer covering of a damaged vein.

Massage of tired varicose veins must be given only by a fully qualified practitioner, because if it is incorrectly performed it can result in breakage of the wall of the vessel.

In the course of this book all these points will be studied in greater detail to enable the reader to grasp the principles of this natural system of healing.

I.
How Varicosity Arises

Most sufferers from this ailment are certain that a fall, accident or some occupation that demands long standing is the cause of the trouble. Examination will show, however, that other people doing exactly the same thing or suffering in the same way are not affected by venous trouble. Certainly there can be exciting causes in this connection, but basically the trouble or weakness arises in the blood stream.

Through wrong food, the choosing of incompatible foodstuffs or inefficient elimination, the blood stream has become thickened, sluggish and acid. This blood, called 'colloidal' in Nature Cure circles, gradually affects the inner wall of the vein and sets up a condition that could be called inflammation. This inflammation is further increased by the acidity of the blood itself, and in due course the muscular tube of the vein becomes weakened. It is then but a short step to varicosity.

When this stage is reached, another factor, the one usually described by the sufferer as causative, comes into play, and this brings about the actual breakage of the vein wall. The second factor may be a severe blow, childbirth, obesity, sudden loss of weight, some twisting or strain of the limb involved such as dislocation of the hip, house-maid's knee, fallen foot arches, some trouble involving the liver or an occupation that demands prolonged standing.

Studying these several causative factors in greater detail, we shall see that in each case there is something that can be done to prevent the formation of varicose swellings.

INJURY
A blow on the fleshy part of the leg should always be treated by rest. It should never be massaged except by an expert masseur, because this can cause rupture of the finer vessels of the injured part. If it discolours badly it should be treated by cold packs and resting, and a crepe bandage should be used to support it until all discolouration disappears. Cold packs and resting are 'safe' treatments and no complications will follow.

PREGNANCY
Most women suffer from enlargement of the veins at this time and it is mainly for this reason that the value of the afternoon rest is so greatly stressed. One or two hours lying with the feet slightly higher than the body is the best possible means of avoiding varicosity of the veins. If this treatment is carried out carefully it will be found that after the baby is born the veins will become quite normal. A balanced dietary with a small amount of protein (eggs, cheese, peas, beans, lentils and milk) and also a small amount of the starchy foods will prevent the liver and bowel from becoming clogged at this time and so choking

the veins. In certain cases it will be found that milk must be restricted in amount because it causes overloading of the stomach. Care in these matters will successfully prevent vein trouble in pregnancy. In Nature Cure circles the value of balanced dieting in pregnancy is stressed because an easy childbirth can then be assured.

CHILDBIRTH

A very heavy baby often results in tearing and prolapse of the vagina and perineal spaces, and this can cause obstruction of the veins and is likely to result in varicosity. This can often be avoided by care during pregnancy. The modern craze which teaches the mother to rise early from the childbed and start exercises often results in prolapse. This again can be prevented if the mother does not hurry her recovery, and one or two more days in bed can often prevent a lifetime of misery. Young mothers should take full advantage of the rest after childbirth and should start abdominal exercises only when they feel vigorous enough to do so without strain. Cold sitz baths and the wearing of cold waist compresses greatly assist in retoning the birth passages.

OBESITY

This is a very common factor in all varicose conditions. Overweight generally means too much fat in the abdomen, with the result that the organs fall and press on the veins as they enter the lower abdomen. A reduction in weight means life in the veins, and all sufferers who are overweight must pay attention to this aspect before they attempt any of the local

measures mentioned later in this book. No quick loss
of weight is desired, but a gradual decrease of two or
three pounds weekly, until a normal weight is
reached, will be sufficient. Abdominal tone can then
be regained by water treatment and graded exercises,
and the organs will regain their normal position.

SUDDEN LOSS OF WEIGHT

It is not generally known that any condition that
brings about a sudden loss of weight can also result in
varicosity. Pathological loss of weight means loss of
fat, and the contents of the abdomen, such as the
intestines, kidneys, bladder and womb, are held in
their place by the fatty tissues. The result of
extensive fat loss is therefore similar to the condition
wherein there is too much fat – in other words,
prolapse or falling of the organs with resultant
pressure on the veins. If, therefore, sudden loss of
weight occurs, abdominal exercises should be practised to ensure that these muscles retain their tone
and keep the lower organs in position, and all efforts
should be made to get weight back to normal by a
balanced dietary.

PELVIC LESIONS

The first injury we think of when the veins of the legs
are involved is some lesion of the pelvic bones. This
trouble is often missed during a diagnostic consul-
tation, except by naturopaths and osteopaths who are
trained to look for such things. A mild dislocation
shows itself by a girdle pain around the lower
abdomen from back to front, and indeed it is often
mistaken for appendicitis. The bladder and bowel also

may be slightly affected. No great force is required to dislocate the pelvis, and a slight twist or fall is often the only history that can be traced. In most cases there is a slight difference in the length of the legs when measured with the patient in a lying position.

If this dislocation is suspected a visit to a competent osteopath or naturopath is advisable, and a few painless manipulations will soon put the matter right. Correction leads to freeing of all the tenseness around the pelvis and to normalization of the flow of venous blood.

HIP DISLOCATION
This is a much more serious trouble and needs immediate attention. Reduction has to be effected under anaesthetic, and X-ray photographs are required to ensure that no permanent injury has been sustained. This is a job for the surgeon.

KNEE INJURY
The most frequent knee injury is a displacement of the cartilages with an escape of fluid which leads to swelling and inflammation of the knee area. If this condition is allowed to progress or to occur frequently, the knee area becomes choked with adhesions and the veins are affected. Osteopathic manipulation of the knee is the best way to treat any recurring displacement of the cartilages, and the services of a trained naturopath or osteopath should always be sought.

FALLEN ARCHES
Finally, in our study of the secondary causes of

varicosity, we come to the feet. No physician can deny that falling of the arches, either frontal or longitudinal, of the feet brings about some twisting of the veins of this part. This leads to tiredness because the venous blood is not withdrawn normally, and loss of tone is increased. Again, correction of such conditions becomes easy when in the hands of a competent naturopath, and many people suffer agony with their feet without ever appreciating the benefits of manipulation.

It must be stressed at this point that very few of the above causes actually bring about varicosity of the veins. The real trouble lies in the condition of the blood and the efficiency of the circulation, and I now propose to take up the former aspect.

2.
Feeding the Veins

To allow nature to effect a cure in any varicose condition two essentials are required. First of all we must ensure that the blood stream is reasonably pure and contains all the mineral salts needed for tissue maintenance, and secondly, that the veins themselves are amply supplied with blood. The methods for the latter condition are described later, and in this chapter I shall describe the type of dietary that makes for a healthy and healing blood stream.

In every diet, raw vegetables must be introduced at least once daily during the winter months and twice daily during the warmer weather. This provision means that the body is supplied in quantity with the mineral salts needed for healthy vein formation. At the same time, vitality in food is also required, and although this is obtained from fresh vegetables, it is also found in fruit. Eat fruit for breakfast or between meals, and try to obtain it as fresh as possible.

Fresh vegetables and fruit are not complete foods, but they give salts and vitamins that ensure the correct working of digestion and the supplying of all tissues with materials that make for real health. They aid assimilation by invigoration of the bowel and also by introducing salts that neutralize acids.

Experience of a large practice proves that if these vital substances are introduced into the diet regularly, the body does not become clogged, and in the case of varicosity the liver is kept lightly loaded and un-hampered. This latter condition is very important because many people suffer from an engorged and sluggish liver, and this immediately causes some back pressure on the veins below and affects them adversely. It is routine Nature Cure treatment in all venous conditions to pay attention to the liver.

Professionally, the liver is first rested by fasting or a complete reduction of the foods that throw strain on the organ. It follows that fatty foods, flesh foods and all forms of oil are completely stopped and that the liver is invigorated by fruit and fruit juices. This treatment results in a reduction of the pressure on the veins and constitutes the first step towards the healing of varicosity.

Certain so-called foodstuffs do not supply the body with usable material but actually deplete the residual supply of mineral salts. If this is continued for years it will be readily understood that the body will never be perfectly healthy. Even the mineral salts introduced in this diet will be insufficient to supply all the tissues. These basically unbalanced foodstuffs are: all white flour products of every description, patent flour, polished rice and all forms of manufactured sugars, tea, coffee and aerated waters. These should be replaced in the diet by wholewheat products, honey or demerara sugar, with dandelion coffee and cereal beverages for drinks.

We are now in a position to arrange a diet that will

greatly aid the treatment of the veins. Such a diet will vary within limits, according to the amount of work done by the sufferer, the assimilative powers and even the time of year, and it must then of necessity be only a rough guide. People doing hard physical work need more starchy food (flour), but in most cases this type of food is largely over-eaten and it must always be taken in as small quantities as possible. Regarding assimilative ability, it is well known that some people can eat large quantities of food and still remain very slim. This means that the bowel is not clean or else it has been damaged in some way (for instance, by colitis) until the area of absorptive surface has been reduced.

SPECIMEN DIETS

In most cases, however, the type of diet outlined will aid this condition by cleansing the bowel and making assimilation of food more efficient. Naturally, more heating foods, namely starches and fats, are required during the cold weather, and an increase in these foods at this time is quite permissible. Always attempt, however, to keep those foods as low as possible, and colds, catarrh and bronchial attacks will be much reduced in consequence.

Breakfast: During the summer months the fresh fruit breakfast is the most cleansing. Apples, oranges, pears, grapefruit, all forms of berries, etc., with a wineglassful of fruit juice such as grapefruit, apple or pineapple. This is naturally a breakfast that is more eliminating than building, but it will aid greatly many people who suffer from vein trouble due to liver congestion.

If it is felt that such a meal does not supply enough heat-giving foods it can be supplemented by dates, figs, raisins, prunes or apricots. Dates supply plenty of sugar for heating and should be taken in limited quantities. The other dried fruits should be soaked for twelve hours and then simmered before being served. This reduces their acidity and makes them slightly alkaline in reaction.

The manual worker will feel that the above type of breakfast is not sustaining enough, and one on the following lines may be substituted, although it is always preferable that a fruit breakfast is taken on one or two mornings weekly.

Some form of whole wheat cereal with a little milk.

Soaked and simmered prunes, figs or raisins.

One or two slices of wholewheat toast or crispbread or oatcake or brown digestive biscuit.

Cup of yeast beverage. (This is a substitute for tea and coffee, which are harmful to the kidneys.)

Lunch: In most cases it is advisable to have some form of vegetable soup. This should be made if possible without meat stock and flavoured with yeast extract. Meat stock soup naturally throws some strain on the liver. Exceptions to the soup course are the people who are very much overweight and whose tissues are already laden with fluid. In such cases the diet should be taken as dry as possible. Liquids only to be sipped when there is actual, compelling thirst.

At this meal a small amount of protein may be introduced. Protein substances build and repair damaged and worn tissues, but their abuse leads to blood and heart conditions. The best proteins in venous troubles are egg, cheese, peas, beans, lentils, nuts, milk and occasionally a little steamed or baked fish. Flesh proteins are best avoided.

Cheese pudding or macaroni and cheese or egg dish or nut dish or vegetarian savoury (made with peas, beans and lentils). With this take a large helping of vegetables and a few potatoes.

Vegetables are best steamed or baked to retain all their strength.

Dessert: Fresh acid fruit is the best after the protein course, but occasionally whole rice pudding or a steamed pudding made from wholewheat flour with dried fruit.

Fresh acid fruit may be taken between meals.

Tea: The last meal is always taken when the body is tired, and in most cases it is preferable to rest for at least twenty minutes before this meal. This allows the digestive tract (especially the liver) to become invigorated and makes digestion of food much easier.

Attention to this little detail often means a great deal to the sufferer from sore or tired legs.

This meal should always be light because this prevents sleepiness just after the meal and does much to ensure a proper night's rest at the normal time. The basis of the evening meal should always be salad, the ingredients depending on the time of year and the substances available.

Small portions of egg, cheese, grated nuts, with a large salad using every kind of vegetable in season such as lettuce, tomato, celery, watercress, onion, turnip, cabbage, carrot, Brussels sprouts, greens, spinach, also dates, figs, raisins, apples, pears and all kinds of tinned fruits.

Wholewheat bread or scone or crispbread or brown digestive biscuit should complete the meal. To those who feel that they need fluid, and to whose constitution it is suitable, China tea, yeast beverage or dandelion coffee is advised.

Supper: If supper is taken it should always be limited to fruit or fruit juices.

FASTING

It was mentioned at the beginning of this chapter that fasting was an ideal way to begin the treatment of varicose conditions, due to its beneficial effect on the liver. Abstention from food gives the whole of the digestive tract a complete rest and healing is then rapid. It will often be found that fasting results in a very coated tongue next morning. This is a sure sign of an engorged bowel and means that the fasting should be prolonged for at least another day and perhaps much longer.

In most cases, however, it is advisable to have prolonged fasting under the care of a trained Nature Cure practitioner who is fully acquainted with the peculiarities of this method of treatment. Many people look askance at this form of cleansing because they are not aware of the benefits, and think that whenever the body is fasted weakness will prevail. This is an old fashioned idea, and many people would obtain a far greater measure of health if they fasted one day weekly.

Without professional advice, it it quite safe for the sufferer from varicosity to fast one day weekly, taking nothing but water. There is no need to rest during this day; indeed, it is usually advisable to be as active as possible, because this aids in the combustion of impurities. The day following the fast the first meal should consist of fresh acid fruits only, because these contain very valuable acids and antiseptics which cleanse the bowel after it has thrown impurities from its wall. If there is no great desire for food after this meal the remaining meals should also be of fruit, and the diet already outlined may be commenced on the third day. There is one important point that must be stressed, and that is the action of the bowel. During the fast day it is likely that it will be quite normal, but during the fruit day it is common to find it is reduced or even missed altogether. This need cause no alarm, because it will regulate itself during the third or fourth day.

The one day fast should be continued at regular intervals. One day each week is most helpful, especially if the patient is very stout and is endeavouring to reduce. In other cases, a fast day once a fortnight is sufficient to keep the bowel cleansing if the rest of the diet is followed carefully.

This diet will gradually supply all the food required to keep the body in health without introducing substances that tend to cause disease. For the actual structure of the veins, however, it is essential that a goodly supply of calcium and fluorine salts is introduced, and stress must be laid on the intake of these salts. Actually they are contained in most vegetables and fruits.

Summary

1. Mineral salts, obtained from vegetables and fruit, are essential to health.
2. In all cases the liver must be rested by proper choice of diet.
3. The diet must be balanced as arranged in this chapter.
4. Fasting is of great benefit when the liver is overworked.

3.
Other Factors

Healing will commence immediately the diet has been started, and I wish now to give you some interesting facts about veins to enable you to follow the cure.

A continuous blood flow is needed for health, and this naturally depends upon the efficiency of the heart, because some eight pints of blood are in circulation in the system. The velocity of flow is greatest near the heart and in the large arteries, but becomes less when the smaller arteries are reached, and in the tiny capillaries it is really quite sluggish, being more of an 'oozing' than an actual flow.

VENOUS FLOW
When the veins are reached, the actual pulsations from the heart are practically lost and venous flow depends on three main factors:

1. The continual following up of the arterial blood into venous spaces.
2. The vacuum created by the pumping action of the heart. This is aided by very deep breathing.
3. The pumping action caused by the expansion and contraction of the muscles surrounding the veins.

People who suffer from varicose veins are conscious of a continual desire to move about to ease the tiredness in the veins, and it is this muscular action that is involved. Blood also flows to the part in which the muscles are being used, and this means that the weakened veins are always getting a good supply of blood which is very beneficial if this blood is in a healthy condition.

In this book we are primarily concerned with the venous system, and therefore we must pay great attention to these vessels, especially those in connection with the lower part of the body and extremities, because it is here that most varicosity occurs.

ABDOMEN

The greatest clusters of veins are found in the abdominal area and in the pelvic cavity. Into these clusters drain the great veins from the legs, and from these the blood goes to the heart. When the abdominal muscles are allowed to sag and the breathing is shallow the veins of the abdomen become engorged and the drainage from the legs is adversely affected. So it is vital in the cure of varicosity that the abdomen be kept in good physical condition.

EXERCISES

The tone of the bowel itself is aided by the diet mentioned, and constipation will be rapidly removed by the roughage involved and also by the stoppage of foods that congest the liver and prevent the natural laxative (the bile) from flowing freely. Deep breathing, by forcing the diaphragm downwards, also brings about an abdominal massage which is extremely beneficial. The following exercises will be most useful.

First Exercise: Stand erect with shoulders drawn back and hands behind back.
Attempt to pull the lowest part of the abdomen inwards and backwards towards the hips. When this is obtained, attempt to lift the abdomen upwards with muscular effort alone. This is a difficult movement to obtain fully, but with practice it will be found that, as the muscle gains strength, the whole abdomen can be lifted upwards. This is the best exercise for middle-aged and elderly sufferers because it can be practised with the least exertion.

Second Exercise: Lying on back with hips high (supported on pillows). Try to bring hips directly over the body, placing the elbows on the floor to aid the support. In this position practise cycling movement, moving the legs as freely as possible. Do this for about twelve movements, and then open and cross the straight legs alternately for the same number. These are the best movements for any kind of abdominal prolapse, and with practice can be done even by the not-so-agile. Properly done, they force the lower abdominal contents high into the upper abdomen and relieve the tension on the upper veins of the legs.

Swollen and knotted veins are not adversely affected by exercise, because muscular movement forces the blood upwards and keeps the veins from becoming overtired. Standing for long periods, or sitting with the knees bent or the legs in a cramped position, does harm to the veins, and it is always a good plan to exercise the toes and feet if forced to stay for a long time in the one position.

BRISK WALKING FOR TIRED VEINS

Brisk walking with the stomach held upward and inward, and practising deep breathing at the same time, is a real tonic to tired veins. This does not mean that you have suddenly to undertake a ten-mile walk. This would only leave the veins tired and strained. Start walking gradually, doing a certain distance each day for a week and increasing it week by week until you are sure that the legs are thoroughly exercised each day. After a walk, alternate spraying of the veins with hot and cold water is most helpful.

RESTING

When the sufferer from varicose trouble is resting he or she should always attempt to get the feet higher than the body. A chair back or some high pillows is ideal for this purpose and, although not dignified, it will be found that this method of assisting drainage will do much to remove the tiredness of varicosity. If desired, the legs can be very lightly massaged in this position. Finger-tip massage is heavy enough and should consist of gently strokings from the ankle towards the body. Heavy massage is dangerous and can further injure the damaged veins.

BANDAGES

There are various theories regarding the supporting of weakened veins by some form of bandage. Many physicians are against this practice because they believe that a supported vein gradually becomes weak and will require continual bandaging. Others think that if the vein is securely supported, the tendency for the trouble to spread is checked.

Undoubtedly there are factors to support both views, because some years ago much damage was done by using very coarse and cumbersome elastic stockings or bandages which caused a great deal of friction on the veins and further damaged them. Veins are extremely sensitive structures and must not be handled roughly or massaged by someone not competent in this art. If, therefore, the condition is not too severe it is advisable to refrain from wearing such supports.

Many people, however, especially those who are overweight and who have to stand for long periods, feel that they must support the damaged vein. Nowadays this support can be obtained by use of thin, fitted elastic stockings which are excellent in every way. Their porous construction allows the skin to breath normally, and since they are washable, cleanliness can be maintained. Therefore, in severe varicosity, relief from pain and tiredness can be obtained from the careful wearing of such stockings. Healing is also aided, provided that extreme care is exercised when the stockings are put on. This should be done before leaving bed in the morning to ensure that the vein has not been allowed to fill with blood before it is supported. Most people find that the removal of the stocking during the resting and sleeping hours prevents cramping of the feet and legs.

Some sufferers cannot get used to the elastic stocking and find that the broad crepe bandage is best. This also has a certain amount of elasticity and can be washed. It is applied just on rising, and it should be wound from the bottom of the leg upwards and fixed with safety pins or tapes. A few days' practice will soon ensure the desired and comfortable tightness of such a bandage. This also should be removed at night.

OXYGEN
The backache and cramp-like pains in the legs that accompany varicosity are really danger signals, warning the sufferer that some form of alleviation is required. Excessive tiredness means a rise in the acidity of the blood. This acid material saturates into the tissues and does not allow the passage of oxygen in sufficient quantities, even if it is introduced, venous sufferers being notoriously shallow breathers. Undoubtedly the lack of oxygen is the originator of the cramping pains, and a reduction in the physical effort of standing, the practice of deep breathing and the protein diet suggested will ease this condition within a very short time.

HIGH HEELS
Much has been written about the detrimental effects of high heels, and certainly, to be really healthy, the body must be kept in a state of skeletal balance.

When the heels are raised two inches from the ground by padding, the weight of the body is thrown forward on the balls of the feet, a part not designed to take most of the weight and absorb the shock of each step. The result is that the entire bony skeleton is jarred with the vibrations of each step, and this alone does much to upset the sensitive nervous system and is an important factor in the growth of nervous diseases.

At the affected joint a great deal of twisting takes place in the veins and arteries, and ultimately this causes some degree of varicosity in the surrounding veins.

Wearing high heels means that the spine just above the hips requires to be thrown forward to preserve balance. The back muscles become contracted, and this causes much of the common back pain experienced by women. The nerves of the spine in this area are also affected, and, as these control the functions of the lower body and limbs and retain the muscular power, many of the common leg troubles arise from this source.

With the throwing forward of the spine, the abdominal contents fall forward on the anterior abdominal wall, causing prolapse and congestion of the bowel, especially when the person becomes overtired or suffers from a serious loss of fat.

AVOID CONSTRICTIONS
It will be easily understood that all forms of constrictions of the surface veins of the legs should be avoided. Garters and suspenders are the main culprits, but tight socks and stockings can also impede the surface circulation of the limbs, and this in turn throws more work on the deeper vessels.

4.
The Water Cure

Once the reader has fully understood the purpose and method of diet it should be gradually introduced. This may take some time, and at first there will be little annoyances because the way the food is arranged may at first cause some digestive upset. When, however, a full Nature Cure diet is firmly established, the patient will feel better, lighter and much more eager to get real health. This feeling of returning health and invigoration must be experienced to be believed, but once appreciated it is seldom that a patient ever returns to the old stodgy type of feeding.

This feeling of aliveness is a sign of returning purity of the blood stream, and it means that this stream can once more perform its real function, that of feeding the tissues and removing from these tissues the debris of metabolism. Now, and not before, is the time to direct the curative effort at the actual damaged vein, because no recovery is possible unless the vein receives an excellent supply of clean blood.

This healing action is achieved in a variety of ways, but undoubtedly the best of all is by the correct use of water. Treatment by water is a science in itself,

and I shall only touch on the fringe of the subject.
Roughly, it is this. When warm or hot water is applied
to the skin surface the arteries and veins dilate and
the blood slows down in its movement. On the other
hand, when cold water is applied to the skin the
arteries and veins contract and the blood moves more
quickly. These are valuable findings and can be
applied with benefit in many cases of ill-health.
Because these water treatments are simple it is
generally supposed that they are old-fashioned, but it
will surprise many people to learn that if there is a
universal cure for all types of ailments it lies in
balanced diet and the *correct use of water externally
or internally.*

HOT AND COLD APPLICATIONS

For swollen veins the reaction of hot and cold water
can be used to increase the blood circulation to the
actual vein wall. It is done in the following manner.
Take two basins, one with hot and the other with
cold water. Apply the water to the skin by way of a
folded towel or pack. The hot pack is first applied as
hot as can be borne for two minutes. It should only
be laid gently on the skin, never being rubbed or
firmly pressed against the vein. Immediately this pack
is removed, apply the cold one, but because the
reaction of cold is so quick this pack should only be
applied for half a minute. Immediately after this
apply another hot pack, and keep doing this alternately for some five or ten minutes. Always finish
with the cold pack.

Such treatment thoroughly removes all debris from
the damaged vein and brings cleansed blood in

abundance – blood which, by virtue of the diet, contains the valuable salts required for healing.

THE COLD SPRAY

If the above treatment can be followed by a cold spray so much the better. A fine spray is best, and the pressure should be so arranged that the leg becomes painful after a few minutes' spraying. This brings about a contraction of the veins, and often badly knotted veins become quite normal in appearance after this application, although this naturally does not last. Of all the local methods the cold spray is undoubtedly the best, being easily applied and having a quick reaction. Any plumber will fit such a spray at a moderate cost, and if connected to the hot and cold taps it can be used for the hot and cold alternate applications and save the trouble of packing.

It is calculated that the reaction of the alternate hot and cold packs is about one hour and that of the cold spray of some two hours' duration. This means that during the rest of the day and night the damaged vein is allowed to work its own cure without aid, and naturally other methods of increasing the power of healing have been sought.

The best of the other methods is the use of cold compresses. These are usually applied at night and kept on during the rest hours. It is not good treatment, however, to keep a local compress working all night, because the slow stimulation of blood tends to bring fresh impurities to the vein when the compress has lost its actual curative effect. To counteract this a waist compress should be worn at the same time, the technique being as follows.

WAIST COMPRESS

Take a piece of linen or cotton material (thin), soak in cold water and apply once round the waist, fastening with safety pins. On no account should two or three layers of cotton be used, as this will prevent the desired temperature from being reached. Cover this wet compress with a layer of flannel or woollen material which should generously overlap the compress. This is applied before retiring and, if need be, a hot water bottle may be used to raise the heat of the body. Normally within a few minutes the desired reaction will be obtained, and by this is meant a feeling of warmth in the compress. This should take place within fifteen minutes. If the compress does not heat it should be removed because the body may become chilled. Usually it will be found that the compress heats for several nights and then the reaction may be poor for a few nights. This is a normal variation and is to be expected.

The local compress is applied at the same time as the waist one. If the veins are on the leg an ordinary bandage is soaked in cold water and wound rather slackly round the affected part of the leg, and this is covered with another crepe bandage or with an ordinary stocking. This combination of waist and leg compress means that increased healing in the damaged part is maintained for a greater part of the night.

The waist compress, in addition to acting as a safeguard for the local application, aids the drainage of the kidneys, invigorates the liver and retones the bowel. It is a most valuable application and is especially useful in cases of liver congestion and haemorrhoids. It should not be applied just before or during the menstrual period.

THE SITZ BATHS

When definite signs of liver congestion are apparent, such as pain beneath the lower right ribs and the appearance of varicose veins in the abdomen, the sitz bath is a very valuable aid. This is actually the old hip bath and is best taken in a bath specially designed for the purpose. Failing this, the ordinary bath will do, and it should be filled as high as possible with slightly warm water. The hips, but not the feet, legs or upper body, are immersed in this bath for about two minutes and then rapidly dried. The best time for this bath is on rising, but many people find it useful before going to bed. If the patient is vigorous, a cold sitz bath may be taken and this will give a very quick and beneficial reaction, stimulating all the abdomen and removing congestion very rapidly indeed. I find these baths most helpful in all conditions of prolapse of the bowel, rectum, womb, and also in liver congestion and haemorrhoids.

The main water treatments to obtain a good result in lower limb varicosity, therefore, should be arranged as follows.

Each morning on rising take the hot and cold spray for a five-minute period followed by a quick cold spray. Two nights weekly the medium-temperature sitz bath should be taken and on the other five nights the waist and leg or local compress should be worn. Such methods ensure that the blood, renewed and vitalized with the foregoing diet, is circulated round the damaged veins.

5.
Constipation

As will be readily understood, constipation is a vital factor in varicosity because the continued presence of faecal matter in the bowel leads to congestion and the large venous clusters in this area become stagnant. This quickly reacts in the lower veins and makes the cure of varicosity impossible until the congestion is lifted.

The regularity of bowel movement varies with each person, and constipation may not be present even when the bowel works every second or even every third day. This also means that the person who has three to five bowel movements each day is not suffering from diarrhoea if such a rhythm is normal to that person.

Constipation is not shown by bowel rate but by other significant signs such as extreme tiredness, lassitude, poor skin with eruptions, offensive breath, mouth and body odour, dirty tongue and muddy complexion. These are all signs of bowel poisoning, and if they are present steps should be taken to activate the bowel more thoroughly.

Once this is decided upon it is usual to think about laxatives and purgatives because these are the general means of cleansing the bowel. Before deciding upon this, however, we must remember that every form of intestinal cleanser acts only because it is an irritant to the bowel, and its forcible expulsion denotes the effort of the body to save itself from further poisoning. Highly vital systems react quickly, but a bowel in poor tone is less sensitive and tends to absorb the poison and harm is ultimately done to the tissues. It is wise, therefore, to regard all purgatives and laxatives as at all times unnatural, to be used as infrequently as possible and then only as a measure extraordinary. The most natural of these laxatives will be found in a strictly herbal group obtainable from Health Food Stores.

ENEMAS

Although the laxative cannot be classified as positive treatment it is not always worse than the enema which is so frequently used in Nature Cure. By such means, water or some fluid is introduced into a part of the bowel designed to receive some fluid only after it has traversed the entire length of the digestive tract. Surely this is more unnatural than the oral intro-duction of laxatives which, after all, are the products of the soil, and in many cases consist of all types of plant. There is, however, a definite place for the plain water enema in the hazards of violent fevers and in cases of extreme bowel decay, but its regular or too frequent use must be deprecated. I will give you one simple rule in this matter. 'When the tongue is deeply coated with fur and the temperature has remained above normal for twelve hours, use the enema.' Avoid it at all other times.

Enemas should always be taken *after* the body has been rested, so they are best taken in the morning after the night's rest. The following technique will give the best results. Lie on the right side on a bed or settee. Let the water flow slowly into the rectum from a gravity-can fixed about three feet above the body. Retain the water and turn over until lying in turn on the back, left side and finally back again to the right side. Retain the water as long as possible before emptying the bowel. If the result is not satisfactory go through the same procedure again. It will usually be found that the plain warm water is sufficient, but if need be a teaspoonful of lemon juice to a pint of water will aid the cleansing.

THE FIRST STEP
A study of physiology proves that after a meal there is a natural relaxation of the muscular sphincter at the end of the bowel. It follows that at this time the bowel is more easily relieved, and it should be a habit to attempt evacuation at this time. No result may come from this habit for the first few weeks, but it must be continued until the body knows that it is being given a chance. Be careful not to overstrain or even spend too long at stool, because these are common causes of rectal prolapse or haemorrhoids.

THE SECOND STEP
Again, physiology teaches that a fluid diet, especially when the fluid is taken before or after a meal, is best for the bowels of people who are inclined to be of a nervous temperament. On the other hand, many people find that if the meals are taken completely

dry, the bowel moves in rhythm. No one can tell which diet will suit and it is a case of trial and error, but if you find that a fluid diet suits you best I should like to give you a word of warning.

Too much fluid, although it may flush the bowel, tends to dilute the blood and weaken the tissues, and stoutness frequently results. So if you find that fluid suits you, keep it up for several months and then gradually reduce the quantity until only a very small amount is being taken. This will ensure that the tissues are kept in good tone and that the bowel is being forced to do some of its own work.

THE THIRD STEP

It is well known that thorough mastication of food and even liquid increases the rate of bowel movement and that people who are inclined to prolonged chewing are seldom constipated. So the person who suffers from bowel sluggishness must chew his food until it is at least semi-fluid before being swallowed. Needless to say, in addition to helping the bowel such methods greatly increase the assimilation of food.

THE FOURTH STEP

Every cure of constipation contains a list of exercises to be performed, and undoubtedly much benefit can be obtained from movement that will increase the muscular power of the abdominal wall.

1. The first exercise is the most important and the simplest. It is brisk walking, keeping the legs as straight as possible and throwing the foot and leg straight forward with each step. A fairly long walk each day will do more to activate the bowel than

any other form of exercise, but it must be practised regularly.

2. The second exercise is also simple. Stand erect and try to raise the leg forward and upward as far as possible. Practise with alternate legs until slightly tired. Remember that throwi the leg upwards is not helpful; it must be lifted by muscular effort.

3. The third exercise is difficult for the beginner but with practice can be easily accomplished. Stand in front of a chair or table with legs slightly apart and the body bent forward, supported by the hands on the table. Completely relax the abdomen. Then with conscious effort, pull the entire contents of the abdomen upwards and inwards, trying to start the movement as low as possible. Continue until slightly fatigued.

These three exercises are all that are required, in conjunction with the foregoing factors discussed, to retone the sluggish bowel.

DIET

The diet of the constipated should contain a large amount of fruit and vegetables because these supply the natural antiseptics of the bowel. The amount of protein and starch should be small, and it will be easily understood that where the bowel action is deficient, all flesh foods should be stopped. The diet advised in this book will be suitable for most cases, although some individual adjustment with regard to the amount of liquid may be required.

6.
Haemorrhoids

This is the term used when the veins of the lower rectum become swollen and varicose. Haemorrhoids can remain active within the confines of the rectum or they can protrude from the opening. In many cases they remain within the rectum until inflammation arises and they then protrude, causing great pain, especially when the bowel is moved. Bleeding from haemorrhoids is common and sometimes reaches serious proportions, causing the sufferer to ultimately become anaemic.

Although an attack of haemorrhoids seemingly comes suddenly, actually it is a condition that develops fairly gradually, and in most cases there is a history of straining at stool, due to constipation. Gradually the lower bowel is forced downwards, and this causes twisting of the veins and the assumption of a swollen appearance. Many women trace this trouble to the birth of a child and undoubtedly this is a common exciting cause, but constipation or weakness of the vein wall has already been present before the birth.

Medical treatment does nothing to remove the real cause of the trouble and consists mainly of injections to wither the pile mass, or, in the event of this not being successful, surgical removal. This latter operation is a painful business and is not always successful, because in many cases the trouble again appears within a year or two.

It will be heartening to sufferers from haemorrhoids to know that, generally speaking, this trouble responds extremely well to Nature Cure treatment. Contrary to medical findings we do not consider the condition really difficult to cure if the patient gives the treatment a fair trial. By this I do not mean that immediate cure is obtainable, because it is likely that several attacks will be experienced after the cure has been commenced. They will gradually become less severe until they only occur after the patient has been indiscreet enough to allow the rectal area to become chilled or has, by eating excessive meals or unbalanced food, allowed the liver to become congested.

The diet already outlined in this book is the basis of the treatment, and it must be kept to as carefully as possible. This light diet removes all strain from the liver within a few weeks. As a result the bile, the natural laxative for a healthy bowel, flows freely and removes constipation, and the congestion of the veins of the rectum is also allayed. Always remember that when you clear your liver and bowel the haemorrhoids will cure rapidly.

If you feel sluggish, easily tired without the expenditure of a great deal of energy; if you experience a heavy, full feeling round the right upper abdomen; if the bowel action is erratic and the stools light in colour; if there is distaste for certain foods which you would normally desire, then you should suspect that your liver is out of order.

There is no need, however, to run for the liver pill or the so-called invigorating liver salts. Nature can cure this condition quickly, efficiently and without upsetting the rest of the digestive tract.

First of all study your own case and also these pointers. The coated tongue and feeling of weight in the abdomen usually mean that you have been overeating proteins. These are eggs, cheese, meat, fish, fowl, peas, beans, lentils and milk. The quickest cure for liver congestion lies in the complete stoppage of these foods until real appetite for them returns, and then they should be limited to the kind advocated in the dietetic part of this book. Always remember that flesh proteins are overrated foods and are at all times dangerous, and that they can easily be replaced by the vegetarian protein with resultant benefit. This applies to manual and mental workers alike, and, contrary to general opinion, it will be found that the vegetarian diet gives greater physical strength to the manual worker.

When the liver area, including the gall bladder, is affected with catarrh, the symptoms are slightly different. There is more sickness and the food is generally distasteful. In this trouble all starchy foods, even of the wholewheat variety, should be reduced to a minimum, and milk and milk foods stopped completely. If severe, every alternate day should be limited to three meals of fresh acid fruit until the condition is completely cured.

The sluggish liver can always be invigorated by deep breathing and side-bending exercises, and in severe cases alternate hot and cold packs, applied to the area around the lower ribs on the right side, will bring relief.

LAXATIVES

Many patients, usually before they fully appreciate the finer points of Nature Cure, ask about a 'good' laxative. The answer is that no laxatives are 'good'. All of them are dangerous, and mostly all of them are not needed. Everything that enters the digestive system is for the purpose of supplying the body with something that has a positive value — in other words, with food. Laxatives and purgatives cannot enter into this class, and rather than acting as a food they could more aptly be described as poisons, although generally of the milder variety.

When a person who has a healthy bowel eats poisoned food the reaction is violent. Diarrhoea, vomiting, sweating, all follow one another in quick succession, and the patient is violently ill, but usually recovers unless he is treated by a scientific doctor who has a remedy for the diarrhoea. Actually diarrhoea is an interesting study, for it shows the main difference between Nature Cure and the allopathic medicine. The naturopath looks upon diarrhoea as a sign that some internal irritation is present and he tries to increase the flow from the bowel. The medical man looks upon it as something he must cure and he does this as quickly as possible thus suppressing the elimination of poisons. Such a patient will usually suffer within a few years from chronic mucous colitis of the bowel, but it will never be suspected that this was the result of poor medication.

No matter what the name on the label, the laxative

or purgative acts as a poison to the human bowel. In health it is a violent reaction, but when the bowel is unhealthy no great disturbance will be noted. This latter is a most serious condition, because it means more and more laxatives will be required to move the poor-toned bowel, and it is not stretching the imagination too far to suspect that some amount of the poisonous laxative will be conveyed through the wall of the bowel into the blood stream.

Therefore, to the healthy, laxatives are always dangerous, but to the possessors of unhealthy sluggish bowels they are absolutely deadly and the strictest care must be exercised in their usage. Every practitioner recognizes that it is sometimes compulsory to give something to stimulate bowel action. In these cases, resort to the most natural of all, such substances as senna or some herbal product, should be made.

WATER TREATMENT

Once the diet has been started and some change of bowel movement recorded, showing that the liver and gall bladder are working more efficiently, local measures can be started in the treatment of haemorrhoids.

If they are internal, a cold sitz (hip) bath should be taken twice weekly. It should be of very short duration, about thirty seconds being sufficient. The reaction should be violent and a feeling of warmth should suffuse the whole body and especially the abdomen. This is easily the best method of toning the abdomen and, combined with the foregoing dietetic advice, will result in a much more efficient circulation of blood through the venous system of the rectum.

EXTERNAL HAEMORRHOIDS

If the piles are external and greatly inflamed, the hot soapy sitz bath is the ideal treatment. Fill a large basin with hot water and add thin shavings of soap, working up a good lather. Immerse the hips completely in this water, trying to work the soapy lather round the pile mass. More hot water should be continually added, and this treatment should be continued for about fifteen minutes. Gradually the irritated sphincter valve at the foot of the rectum will relax and the pile mass can be gently eased into the rectum. This may occur during the first hot sitz bath, but generally when the inflammation is severe two or even three baths will be required before the piles can be reintroduced into the rectum.

Once this is accomplished the part should be bathed with cold water or else the hips immersed in cold water for about thirty seconds. After this, an occasional quick cold sitz bath will ensure that the pile mass does not again protrude.

When there is a tendency to piles it will easily be understood that all chilling of the rectum must be avoided and that it is unwise to sit on cold surfaces. If this has been unavoidably done the hips should be immersed in hot water as soon as possible. All cold water bathing should be avoided by women at the menstrual period.

7.

Phlebitis

At the start of this book I stated that varicosity originated with slight and seemingly unimportant inflammations on the inner walls of the veins near the valves. These inflammations are usually painless and pass unnoticed except in certain cases where a venous weakness is already present. Most people, however, are not aware of them, and years elapse before vein swelling shows that the valves have been damaged.

When the inflammation becomes acute, however, the condition is called phlebitis and it can develop into serious trouble if it is not correctly treated. The danger here lies in the tendency for a part of the inflamed valve to break away and work its way into the venous system and choke some blood vessel at a distant part of the body. This can be prevented by careful treatment provided it is conducted along the lines suggested in this chapter.

Phlebitis shows itself by pain, stiffness, and inflammation of a part along the course of the vein, usually of the leg. The condition quickly generalizes and the sufferer is physically upset. The damaged part then becomes red with a certain degree of burning and swelling, and the need to rest the leg becomes essential.

TREATMENT

The part should be bathed with hot and cold water. This is best done by using two cloths, one for hot and the other for cold. Lay the hot cloth gently on the part and keep it on for two minutes. Then apply the cold one for half-a-minute. Continue in this way alternately for fifteen minutes, always finishing with the cold application. This treatment should be used four or five times daily when the condition is acute. No pressure or any form of massage should be used on the painful spot.

Between the hot and cold treatments the limb should be rested as much as possible, and it is greatly eased if it can be supported slightly higher than the rest of the body. This is especially valuable in young or middle-aged people, but it is not so advisable in the elderly because there is always the danger of chest congestion if they lie too long in the resting position.

While resting, a cold wet pad of linen should be applied over the inflamed area. Next to this place oil silk, a thick pad of cotton wool, and a bandage which should be applied very loosely.

These are the ideal local measures but they can be greatly aided by attention to the diet. The underlying cause of phlebitis is the same as that of all varicose conditions, namely some form of toxaemia in the blood. Every effort must be made at this time to cleanse the blood, and by far the safest and quickest way to do this is by fasting. Stop all food and liquid except water, which should be taken when there is actual thirst. This means that the energy used for digestion is not needed, and when combined with complete physical rest it gives the body the greatest opportunity to cleanse the blood and start healing. The fast may be continued for up to five days, depending upon the amount of inflammation present. Normally, it would not be stopped until the part is very much better, because immediately food is taken the rate of healing is very much reduced, but it is unwise to undertake a long fast without professional supervision.

During the fast it is likely, because toxaemia is always present, that the tongue will be very dirty, and if this reaches serious proportions the warm water enema (described in another chapter) should be used for one or two mornings. This aids the condition and makes for more rapid healing, but it should only be used in very dirty conditions.

When the healing has so progressed that the inflammation is rapidly subsiding, the fast should be broken with fruit. Take acid fruit such as apples, oranges, pears, grapes, grapefruit, with apple, orange or grapefruit juice for one or two days before starting on the general diet advised in this book. Fresh acid fruit is very antiseptic and, when taken immediately after a fast, cleanses the bowel and ensures rapid assimilation of food.

From all this it will be understood that phlebitis is in the nature of a warning on the part of the body. It shows that there is an impurity within the blood stream and also that the condition of the veins is below par. Heed the warnings and you will attain health.

8.
Varicose Ulcers

This distressing and painful condition affects large numbers of sufferers, and many and varied are the methods of alleviation. Ointments and special types of bandages are widely used, some with success but others with greatly disappointing results. Generally speaking, a discharging ulcer is most difficult to heal, and better results are always obtained if the skin is just cracked and there is no discharge.

The reason for this lack of success by such methods is easily explainable by Nature Cure theory. In such cases it is understood that there is within the body some impurity, usually the result of unbalanced dietary, but often from the partaking of drugs and pain-killers. This impurity should normally be eliminated through such channels as the liver, bowel, skin, kidneys and lungs, but these patients have reached such a poor state of bodily health that their organs are unable to deal adequately with the large amount of harmful material.

What happens then is easily understandable. The body in both health and disease will always attempt to cleanse itself, and in the case of varicose ulcer there is first of all a weakness in the veins. Eventually these are forced to burst, and the body pours its impurity through this channel. Whenever this occurs there is some germ invasion, and the part becomes nauseous and evil-smelling.

From one point of view the varicose ulcer is a good thing because it relieves the body of impurity which must eventually kill, and I have known cases that, wrongly treated by suppressive methods, terminated fatally within a few short months. Ideally the varicose ulcer should heal without aid. That is true healing, and the methods outlined in the foregoing part of this book should form the basis of all such treatment. Get the body into a healthy state, and allow it to cleanse as much as possible. Then, when the amount of residual impurity within the body, always present due to our eating habits, reaches a normal level, the varicose ulcer will heal beautifully by first intention.

This method of treating such obstinate conditions is impressively successful provided the patient fully understands exactly what is taking place and aids and abets the cure.

Now let us take the case of a discharging varicose ulcer which has been treated by suppressive ointments without effect and which is gradually enlarging in its area and increasing in its degree of pain.

The first treatment is to wash round the wound with warm soapy water and apply a plain bandage with a layer of vaseline. No other ointment is to be used and no drugs of any kind are to be taken. The bandage should be removed and changed several times during the day, and the part bathed at the same time with warm soapy water. The external bandage should be of porous material and naturally the painful part should be protected against injury, but there is no harm in exposing it to the air or sun for a short period each day. The use of an artificial sun lamp is to be recommended. When this is done we leave the actual ulcerated part severely alone.

Now we turn our attention to the cleansing of the body, and the best way to begin this is with a short fast. One to three days without food (longer if very much overweight) is sufficient to start the treatment. Take plenty of water and rest if you feel tired, although it is possible to continue at fairly hard work for the first two days of a fast. During the fast, here is what will usually happen to you. First of all you will feel hungry, often light-headed and usually during the first night will be troubled with a headache. Next morning your tongue will be coated and this should give you some indication of the internal condition of the bowel. During the second day you will still feel hungry and water should be taken freely. The headache will not be so bad but you will likely feel squeamish and your tongue will still be coated. On the third morning the tongue will still be dirty, in fact the coating may be much thicker, and the breath will be heavy. This day, however, you will feel better and lighter and generally more able to do things, and as the fast proceeds you will feel the general invigoration of your body becoming cleaner. At first, however, the three days' fast is long enough, and you should break it on the fourth day.

BREAKING FAST
The best way to break the fast is by taking nothing but fruit on the first day. The best kinds are

grapefruit, oranges, apples, pears and plums, because these supply antiseptic substances which remove the debris of the cleansed bowel. After this the diet advocated in the foregoing part of this book should be commenced and very strictly adhered to for a lengthy period. Ideally several of these fasts should be taken to increase the cleansing. Some people find that a three-day fast each month does them a great deal of good but others prefer to have a one-day fast each week, because they find that the longer fast does not agree with them. In both cases the acid fruit day should always follow.

In Nature Cure circles most people take plain warm-water enema after a fast to wash away accumulated impurities. I do not believe this is necessary in such short fasts, and generally it will be found that the bowel will regulate itself after the fruit day. When you are on a meatless diet it really does not matter whether the bowel works perfectly or not, because no decaying matter is introduced and the bowel will naturally find its own rhythm.

This fasting and dieting should be continued for eight weeks, and during all this time no other treatment except the vaseline pad should be applied to the varicose ulcer. If the veins of the leg are swollen they may be subjected to the water treatment advised, but the actual ulcer should be treated with the warm water bathing and the vaseline pad. The discharge will vary considerably with the dieting. Some days it will be less profuse and on others it will run freely. The type of discharge also varies from day to day. The body, given this golden opportunity to cleanse, will make full use of the wound and it must be left to work its own salvation.

Between the sixth and eighth weeks there will generally be a positive cleansing upset in which the body makes a determined effort to rid itself of impurity. Generally, the patient feels sluggish and without appetite and the wound may be very active. A fast is always indicated at this stage and should be continued until the desire for food returns, when at least one day on fruit should be taken. This upset is a very good sign, because it means that the body is regenerating and finding some of its lost health. In most cases it is not severe and need cause no great inconvenience, and if properly treated will leave the patient refreshed and invigorated.

LOCAL MEASURES
It is usual to find that after the crisis the ulcer shows definite signs of healing. The discharge becomes less nauseous, and healing is seen round the edges of the wound. At this stage the following local measures will bring about a rapid change in the condition.

Obtain a good piece of thin linen, boil it thoroughly and cut a small hole in the middle. Then cut it to a size just a little larger than the wound. Soak in cold water and apply wet to the wound. This linen is never removed until the wound is competely healed unless it is extra large, when another piece may have to be cut. The hole in the linen is to allow the discharge to come away freely. Cover this linen with a damp cloth and never allow the linen to dry, by keeping this upper cloth always wet. At first this application will bring about a great soothing, but gradually a little heat will be found in the wound and it will become itchy, always a good sign of healing. Keep continually changing the damp cloth to allow the wound to heal in moist heat. Actually the linen will fall off when the wound is healed, but each day a little can be cut off with scissors to prevent it from catching on the damp cloth.

This wet-cloth technique is very effective, but only after the diet has been adhered to and the other methods have been used to stimulate the venous circulation. It is useless to try to cure a varicose ulcer by means of this application alone, because the body is still full of impurity and then it becomes a suppressive treatment very much akin to that of ointments.

TWO CASE HISTORIES

Here are two examples of the efficacy of such treatment. In the first case an elderly man suffered from a terrible leg ulcer which had practically stripped the flesh from knee to ankle. He had tried every method possible and had even gone to Paris and New York to receive special treatment which proved successful for only a limited time and then the leg became as bad as ever. When the above scheme was suggested he was sceptical, but after persuasion decided to give it a trial. The diet was started gradually without fasting because he was in a very weakened condition. At the same time a small waist compress was worn and the leg compressed above the knee where the various veins were enlarged.

Gradually the diet took effect and the patient was able to leave his bed and take some exercise, mainly short walks. No other application was used on the ulcer except vaseline pads, although occasionally olive oil was applied. The discharge from the leg was profuse and the wound painful. About ten weeks after the treatment was commenced the patient contracted a severe cold and was fasted for several days, the fast being concluded with a fruit day. During the cold, all discharge from the wound ceased, rather an unusual occurrence, but it again commenced after the cold had cleared. About a week after the cold, the wet application was first used, the whole of the foreleg being covered. The wound was so large that during the first week the linen had occasionally to be removed because the healing pain was so intense. This is not common in smaller ulcers. Gradually, however, the pain became quite bearable and each time I visited the patient I was able to cut away quite a lot of the linen. The last part to heat was a point just above the ankle which discharged for a long time and then healed completely within a few days. After this the healed part was treated for a fortnight by cold spraying and then all treatment was stopped. The diet was kept up and now, years afterwards, the patient is still keeping to balanced meals and has never had the slightest trouble with the leg.

CLEANSING THE BOWEL

In the second case, both the legs were affected, although the ulceration was not so extensive as in the above. The patient had a long history of allopathic treatment without any real improvement, and when she first visited me one leg was encased in an elastic bandage. This bandage had to be worn for several weeks at a time. The cure was commenced in much the same way as for the previous patient, but very little attention was paid to the legs at first. The patient had been using zinc ointments, and when these were stopped the skin over the wounds became very thick and scaly. Slight leakages appeared in this scaly mass, but except for occasional soapy compresses the wounds were left alone.

Diet started with a two-day fast when it became obvious that the patient's bowel was in a very unwholesome condition. A vegetable and fruit diet was then prescribed, and after three weeks she developed a form of mucous colitis which greatly helped in the cleansing of the bowel. A fruit diet was given at this time and continued for another week, when the colitis cleared up. The patient was then advised a diet along the lines of the general one advocated in this book, and it soon became obvious that she was going to make a good recovery. Her weight came down fairly rapidly, about three pounds weekly, and she looked fitter and younger in every way.

Three months passed and it still seemed that the legs were not making much headway although the patient felt very well indeed. About this time another bout of mucous colitis developed and it lasted about a fortnight. It was treated mainly with fruit and warm sitz baths and again left the patient fresher and healthier. Shortly after this the thickened skin of the legs began to disperse, revealing a beautiful healthy skin formation beneath, and this continued until healing was complete.

These are commonsense methods of treating

varicose ulcers: attacking the cause, cleansing the blood and then allowing the body to do its own healing with only a little aid to speed the progress. By such simple means great benefit will be achieved by all who suffer in this way.

Conclusion

By this time the reader will appreciate that although I have diverged occasionally to describe specific troubles the main theme of this book is that the body, given proper chance, will always attempt to cure itself of venous troubles and indeed of all other troubles.

Disease arises from three main causes. The first is negative thinking, a profound weakness in our race perhaps traceable to our somewhat mystical forbears who in their ignorance thought it was calling down a judgement to think and look outward. This aspect is thoroughly dealt with in the many splendid magazines and books on psychology, and it is outside the scope of our present subject.

The second is the taking of impoverished and unbalanced food which does not supply the body with the material actually required for its maintenance and to replace the wear and tear in the tissues. Actually in this country we all need a very plentiful supply of balanced vegetables to equalize our large starch intake which is required to combat the cold weather. Starch poisoning is perhaps the greatest danger and its detrimental effects can be greatly controlled by an abundance of vegetables and fruit. Wholewheat starch is better than white, an important factor amply proved during the war, but it also must not be overeaten. The proteins are the most detrimental foods to the liver and they must be taken in moderation because health in the liver means health in the body. If the diet is composed of twenty per cent protein, twenty per cent starch and the rest of fruit, vegetables, sugars and fats, health can easily be maintained.

The third cause of ill-health is inefficient elimination. This is generally connected with bowel action, but actually the workings of the skin, lungs, and kidneys are equally as important. Air and sun baths with friction rubs keep the skin healthy, deep breathing ensures lung movement and the curtailment of harmful liquids allows the kidneys to do their own work with plenty of reserve.

All these points are important if we are to maintain and regain health and, combined with the major points explained in this book, they will do much to cure completely any case of vein weakness.

Have you read these best selling ABOUT books?

ABOUT GINSENG

This book tells how ginseng has been used as a panacea for thousands of years in the East, describes its natural habitat and its cultivation throughout the world, and gives scientific evidence of its properties — especially its effect on the ageing process. The author reviews the different forms available and gives advice on how best to take it.

ABOUT VITAMINS

In this age of processed foods it is becoming increasingly more important to ensure that our diets provide us with an adequate supply of vitamins for the maintenance of good health. This book, an introduction to the subject of vitamins, clears away any misunderstandings that might exist, and tells the fascinating story of man's discovery of nature's keys to radiant health.

ABOUT RAW JUICES

The juices of fresh fruit and vegetables play a vital part in restoring and maintaining optimum health, and this book shows you how to select, prepare and use such life-giving and delicious drinks both for fortification against disease and for the specific treatment of certain ailments.

ABOUT GARLIC

Gives the historical background to this amazing herb, and shows how its miraculous healing powers can protect your health and assist the cure of many and varied complaints. The book also contains hints on the use of garlic in the kitchen, and recipes are included for garlic flavoured dishes.